Better Health with a Drink
(Journey to a better you)

By: Audriana Woods

Healthy eating is a part of our living to ensure that our bodies are getting the right amount of nutrition. Many people are looking for something so simple and easy to do to help lose weight and become healthier. I have researched so many easy ways to lose weight and I have found several other ways to start off especially if you are not able to go to the gym. Detoxed are trending now that are used to help start off with losing weight and killed the toxins in the body.

Here is a quick list of detox drinks to help with losing weight and gaining nutrition back into your body.

- **Cucumber, lemon, and lime water**
  - Empty half gallon drinking container
  - 2 lemons
  - 2 limes
  - 1 cucumber
    - Sliced the lemons, limes, and cucumber
    - Placed them into the container
    - Filled container with water
    - Let sit for 2 hours or 24 hours for better results

  - Boosting your immune system
  - Cleaning how horrible toxins
  - Anti-inflammatory
  - Helps you to stay hydrated

- **Strawberry and tangerine water**
  - Empty half gallon drinking container
  - Half a cup of strawberries
  - 1 tangerine
    - Peeled and sliced tangerine
    - Sliced strawberries in half
    - Placed them into the container
    - Filled container with water
    - Let sit for 2 hours or 24 hours for better results
  - High in vitamin C
  - Metabolism boosters

- **Mint, blueberries, and raspberries water**
  - 4 tbsp. of mint
  - Half of cup of blueberries
  - Half of cup of raspberries
    - Chopped mint
    - Sliced blueberries in half
    - Sliced raspberries in half
    - Placed them into the container
    - Filled container with water
    - Let sit for 2 hours or 24 hours for better results

- o High in vitamin C
- o Help boost immune system
- o Mint helps with the detox

If you are much of a water drinker here are some tea recipes that with knock your metabolism in high gear.

- **Cayenne tea**
    - o ¼ tsp-1 tbsp of cayenne pepper
    - o 8 oz of warm or hot water
        - 8 oz of warm/hot water
        - Mixed the amount of cayenne pepper with warm/hot water
        - I recommend twice a day
- **Green tea with Cayenne pepper and honey**
    - o 1 pouch of pure green tea
    - o ¼ tsp of cayenne pepper
    - o ¼ tsp of honey
        - 8 oz of warm/hot water
        - Mixed cayenne pepper and honey with warm/hot water
        - I recommend twice a day

Another item that helps with weight loss is Bragg's Apple Cider Vinegar (raw and unfiltered). This brand was found to be the most effective when it came to weight loss. Here are a couple of recipes that I have used to continue my weight loss journey and for those who are always on the go.

- **Apple Cider Special**
    - o 1 tsp of ACV
    - o 1 tsp of lemon juice
    - o 8 oz of warm water
        - I recommend drinking this about twice a day
- **Apple Cider Delight Smoothie**
    - o 1 tsp of ACV
    - o 1 cup of strawberries
    - o 1 cup of orange juice
    - o 1 ½ cup of ice
        - Mix everything in a blender
- **Apple Cider Tea**
    - o 1 tsp of ACV
    - o 1 tbsp of honey
    - o 1 bag of green tea
        - I recommend drinking this before going to bed.
- **Apple Cider Citrus Tea**
    - o 2 cups of water
    - o 2 tbsp of ACV

- 1 grapefruit, sliced in fours
- 1 orange, sliced in fours
- 1 lemon, sliced in fours
- A small piece of ginger root
- 3 tbsp of honey
- 1 bag of green tea
    - Mix all the ingredients together in a pot until it comes to a boil then add the green tea bag.
    - Allow to sit for about 3 minutes, so the flavors can settle together.
- I recommend at any time and its great as Iced Tea.

JOURNEY TO A BETTER YOU

A mini journal to track on your progress for short or long-term goals with a healthier you.

Health Tips:
(1) Have at least 8 hours of sleep.
(2) Do not have a worry or stressful mind before going to sleep.
(3) Drink 8 cups of water a day
(4) If you can, avoid using the elevator and take the stairs.
(5) Throughout the day, snack on fruits and veggies.
(6) Do not eat after 7:30 pm/ Do not eat an hour before going to sleep.
(7) Eat light for dinner

Spiritual Motivation (NIV):
(1) 1 Cor. 6:19-20: "Do you not know that your bodies are temples of the Holy Spirit, who is in you, whom you have received from God? You are not your own; you were bought at a price. Therefore, honor God with your bodies."
(2) 3 John 1:2: "Dear friend, I pray that you may enjoy good health and that all may go well with you, even as your soul is getting along well."
(3) 1 Cor. 10:31: "So whether you eat or drink or whatever you do, do it all for the glory of God."
(4) 1 Tim 4:8: "For physical training is of some value, but godliness has value for all things, holding promise for both the present life and the life to come."
(5) Jer. 33:6: "Nevertheless, I will bring health and healing to it; I will heal my people and will let them enjoy abundant peace and security."
(6) Pro, 16:24: "Gracious words are a honeycomb, sweet to the soul and healing to the bones."
(7) Pro. 3:7-8: "Do not be wise in your own eyes; fear the Lord and shun evil. This will bring health to your body and nourishment to your bones."